Wafa Dahmani
Nour Elleuch
Hanène Jaziri

Celiac disease and quality of life

Wafa Dahmani
Nour Elleuch
Hanène Jaziri

Celiac disease and quality of life

ScienciaScripts

Imprint
Any brand names and product names mentioned in this book are subject to trademark, brand or patent protection and are trademarks or registered trademarks of their respective holders. The use of brand names, product names, common names, trade names, product descriptions etc. even without a particular marking in this work is in no way to be construed to mean that such names may be regarded as unrestricted in respect of trademark and brand protection legislation and could thus be used by anyone.

Cover image: www.ingimage.com

This book is a translation from the original published under ISBN 978-620-6-72513-8.

Publisher:
Sciencia Scripts
is a trademark of
Dodo Books Indian Ocean Ltd. and OmniScriptum S.R.L publishing group

120 High Road, East Finchley, London, N2 9ED, United Kingdom
Str. Armeneasca 28/1, office 1, Chisinau MD-2012, Republic of Moldova, Europe
Printed at: see last page
ISBN: 978-620-0-30336-3

Contents

1 INTRODUCTION

Celiac disease (CD) is an autoimmune enteropathy caused by intestinal inflammation triggered by gluten ingestion in gënëtically prëdisposedës(1).

Its clinical presentation is protëiform, its classic picture of chronic diarrhoea with a deficiency syndrome being supplanted by a wide range of digestive and extra-digestive manifestations of the most disturbing kind(2).

Once considered a rare disease, CD is now recognised as a common condition, affecting around 1% of the world's population (3).

In Tunisia, there is a lack of epidemiological data on CD, which suggests a prevalence of around 0.7% in adults (4) and between 0.5 and 1% in children (5). Moreover, some studies suggest that its prevalence is similar to that observed in other Mediterranean countries, varying between 0.3 and 0.6% (6).

It can occur at any age, with two peaks in frequency: in children aged between 6 months and 2 years, and in adults aged between 30 and 40 years (7). The male/female sex ratio is 1:2 to 4, with a predominance of females generally reported (8,9).

Treatment of CD remains exclusively dietetic, based on a strict gluten-free diet (GFD) for life (10).

Its prognosis depends mainly on the development of complications, in particular osteoporosis and malignancy, which occur in most cases due to poor adherence to the GFR (11-13).

Because of its symptoms on the one hand, and because of the constraints associated with GVHD on the other, CD can have a considerable impact on patients' quality of life (14). Indeed, the various manifestations that can accompany this disease, from chronic diarrhoea to iron-deficiency anaemia and unexplained primary sterility, can have a major impact on the daily lives of patients with CD. This is all the more true given that the disease is often diagnosed late, months or even years after the onset of symptoms. Adherence to the GFD can also prove restrictive and have a considerable impact on the quality of life of celiacs. The need to follow a strict gluten-free diet may not only largely limit patients' food choices, but also limit opportunities for socialising around meals, thus impacting their social life which could in turn alter patients' psychological balance (15,16). In addition, the higher cost of gluten-free foods and the need to constantly check product labels can add an extra financial and mental burden to patients. These factors combined may contribute to a significant alteration in the QoL of patients with CD.

Thus, assessment of QoL during CD is of major importance. It is a means not only of assessing the impact of the disease, but also of promoting the patient's collaboration in the management of his or her condition, possibly leading to better compliance with the GMP.

Numerous questionnaires concerning quality of life exist, some of which are specifically intended for celiac patients. These specific questionnaires would make it possible to highlight the different areas of QoL impacted by CD, as well as the intensity of their impact on patients' lives.

To our knowledge, no Tunisian study has been carried out on this subject in celiac patients.

It is with this in mind that we have proposed, through this work, to :

> Assessing HRQoL during CD.

> To determine the factors associated with impaired QoL in patients with CD.

2 MATERIALS AND METHODS

1. TYPE OF STUDY :

This is a cross-sectional study with an analytical purpose, ëtalëe over a 3-month period from October to 31 December 2023.

2. STUDY POPULATION :

2.1. CHOICE OF POPULATION

We chose as our target population the members of the Association Tunisienne de la Maladie Creliaque (ATMC) in order to have a representative sample in terms of numbers and regional distribution. This is the only national association with more than 6,000 members from all regions of the country. Prior telephone agreement was obtained from the association's president.

2.2. INCLUSION CRITERIA :

Included in our ëtude were patients:

> Over 18s.

> Consent.

> Known carriers of CD for at least 12 months (Hëbl! minimal jugë necessary to be able to assess the impact on daily life).

The diagnosis of CD is self-reported and previously confirmed on the basis of serological and histological evidence for all members of the ATMC.

2.3. NON-INCLUSION CRITERIA :

Patients were not included in our study:

> Suffering from a serious chronic illness that can have an impact on quality of life (chronic renal failure, cirrhosis, heart failure).

2.4. EXCLUSION CRITERIA :

Patients were excluded from our study:

> Did not complete the entire questionnaire.

3. DATA COLLECTION :

The data was collected using a digital questionnaire on the Google forms platform.

The questionnaire was distributed by email from 01/10/2023. The e-mail addresses of the target patients were obtained by contacting them through the official ATMC group on the Facebook social network.

Two reminders were subsequently sent on 01/11/2023 and 01/12/2023.

The questionnaire consisted of 55 questions, completed in around 08 minutes. It was divided into 3 parts, as follows:

3.1. FIRST PART :(ANNEX I)

The first part of the questionnaire concerned the socio-demographic, anamnestic and clinical characteristics of the patients, including :

3.1.1. Socio-demographic characteristics :

> Age

> The genre

> Living environment: urban or rural

> Educational level: primary, secondary or university education

> Marital status: single, married, divorced or widowed.

> The socio-economic level (NSE).

3.1.2. Lifestyle habits :

> Smoking

3.1.3. Pathological antecedents and comorbidities:

> Familial anteëcëdents (ATCD) of CD

> Personal history of autoimmune diseases associated with CD.

3.1.4. History of the disease :

> The age of discovery of CD.

> The duration of the disease.

3.2. Part Two:

The second part of the questionnaire was devoted to assessing adherence to the GFD. In order to have an objective evaluation, we used a valid score to classify patients according to their level of adherence to the GFD: the ***BiagiGluten-free diet compliance score (Biagi score)* (Appendix II)**.

3.3. PART THREE :

> The last part was dedicated to QoL assessment.
To do this, we used two valid questionnaires in Arabic:

> A generic questionnaire: the SF-12 **(Appendix III)** .

> A specific questionnaire: the Creliacdisease questionnaire (CDQ**) (Appendix IV)**.

4. OPERATIONAL DEFINITION OF VARIABLES :

4.1. The socio-economic level :

An NSE is considered low, medium or high depending on the household's monthly income:

> Low if income is < 500 Tunisian dinars (TND) per month.

> Medium if income is between TND 500 and 1500 per month.

> Hleve if income > TND 1,500 per month.

4.2. Le Biagi score :

It is a validated score based on a questionnaire which evaluates the strategies used by patients to avoid all involuntary ingestion of gluten (17,18). It provides a final score in five levels (0 - IV), which, from a clinical point of view, can be grouped into three levels as follows:

> *0 and I*: No follow-up by the RSG

> Π : Follow-up of the RSG but with significant errors that need to be corrected

> *Het W*: Strict monitoring of the RSG.

4.3. THE SF-12 :

This questionnaire is the short version of the SF-36 (19). It consists of 12 questions, divided into 8 dimensions, each corresponding to a different aspect of health:

> Physical activity

> Social life

> Physical pain

> General health lost

> Vitality

> Limitations due to mental state

> Limitations due to physical condition

> Mental health

These dimensions are combined to calculate two sub-scores:

> A physical HRQoL sub-score.

> A mental HRQoL sub-score.

The overall score and each of the sub-scores range from 0 to 100.

A score of less than 40 defines an altered HRQoL for the dimension in question (20).

In this study, we used the Arabic version of the questionnaire after obtaining the author's agreement (21).

4.4. THE CDQ :

This is a self-administered questionnaire for assessing the QOL of patients with CD devised by Hauser et al. in 2007 (22). It consists of 28 questions to assess 4 domains:

> Emotions.

> Social problems.

> Gastrointestinal symptoms.

> Worries (related to the illness and the GSR)

Each domain comprises seven questions, each scored on a Liekert scale from 1 to 7. The score for each area varies from 0 to 49 points, with a total score between 0 and 196.

The lower this score, the more the QoL is altered.

To date, no clear threshold has been established to dichotomise CDQ scores.

We used the Arabic version of the questionnaire, validated in a Moroccan population; the author's agreement was obtained beforehand (23).

5. STATISTICAL ANALYSIS OF DATA :

The data *was* entered and analysed using SPSS software version 26.0.

5.1. DESCRIPTIVE STUDY :

Frequencies and percentages were calculated for qualitative variables, as well as means, standard deviations, medians, interquartile range [25th percentile-75th percentile] and range of extreme values for quantitative variables, according to the normality of these variables.

5.2. ANALYTICAL STUDY :

❖ Univariate analysis:

> To compare two means, the Student's t-test was used for quantitative variables that follow a normal distribution and are homogeneous. When the distribution is not normal, the comparison was made using the U-Man-Whitney test.

> To compare percentages, we used the Chi-square test if all the theoretical numbers were greater than or equal to 5, and Fisher's exact test, in the case of a study of the relationship between two binary qualitative variables with at least one calculated theoretical number less than 5.

> The link between 2 quantitative variables was studied using Pearson's correlation coefficient. The correlation coefficient 'r' varies from -1 (negative correlation: the higher one variable is, the lower the other is, and vice versa) to +1 (the higher one variable is, the higher the other is, and vice versa), passing through zero = no correlation. The significance corresponds to the "p": if $p < 0.05$, then the "r" is significantly different from zero: so, depending on whether it is positive or negative, there is a positive correlation or a statistically significant negative correlation. In all statistical tests, the significance level has been set at 0.05.

❖ The association between the explanatory variables and the variations in the various scores (total score, scores in each domain) was verified using the latter as continuous quantitative variables.

❖ **Multivariate analysis :**

> Factors with a p-value <0.2 in the univariate analysis were included in the multivariate models, where linear regression was used to identify factors associated with HRQoL, taking into account confounders.

6. BIBLIOGRAPHIC RESEARCH :

We conducted a bibliographic search of the Cochrane, Google Scholar, Pubmed and Science Direct global digital library databases. The most frequently used keywords were: Celiac disease, impact, gluten-free diet, quality of life.
We have used Zotero to manage the references we have chosen.

7. WRITING THE THESIS :

For the writing of the thesis, we adopted the IMRAD format for scientific writing as well as the recommendations of the Thesis Committee of the Faculty of Medicine of Sousse.

8. Ethical considerations :

This study was тепёе in compliance with ethical standards in research, namely 1 anonymity and confidentiality of data. Indeed, the personal data collected in the questionnaire did not allow the speaker to be identified as a natural person, either directly or indirectly. The collection of this data was therefore not subject to a protective legal framework.

Informed consent was obtained from all participants in the study by including a "consent" question in the questionnaire after a detailed explanation of the interest and protocol of the study.

Professional medical confidentiality was respected.

The results of this study will be used for scientific purposes only.

3 RESULTS

1. **DESCRIPTIVE STUDY**

1.1. WORKFORCE :

Out of **190** patients contacted, **135** completed the questionnaire.

Of these, **31** patients were not ële included, distributed as follows:

> 11 did not consent to take part in the study.

> 7had other chronic pathologies that could interfèrer with the results.

> 13 were under the age of 18.

Four patients were excluded for not completing the questionnaire in full.

In the end, our study involved 100 patients.

Figure 1 illustrates theflow chart of the study

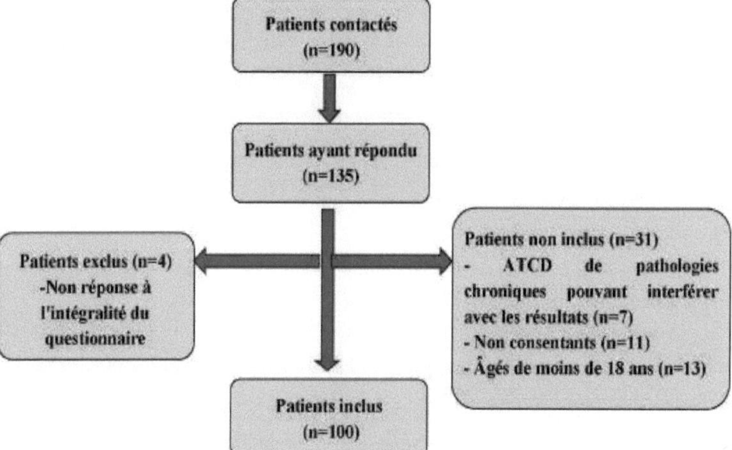

Figure 1: Flow diagram of the study.

1.2. **EPIDEMIOLOGICAL AND DEMOGRAPHIC CHARACTERISTICS**

1.2.1. Age :

The mean age of patients ël.ай 34.5 ± 9.5 years with extremes ranging from 18 to 62 years.

The age group most represented ëwas between 26 and 35 (41%) (Figure 2).

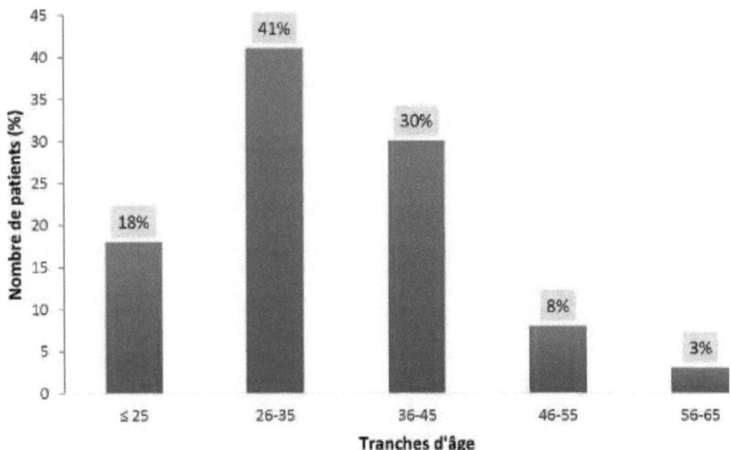

Figure 2: Distribution of patients according to age

1.2.2. Genre:

Our population was predominantly female (72%) with a sex ratio (male/female) of 0.39.

1.3. SOCIO-ECONOMIC CHARACTERISTICS :

1.3.1. Marital status :

Fifty patients (50%) were single, 44 (44%) were married. We also included 5 patients (5%) who were divorced and one widowed patient (1%).

1.3.2. Socio-economic level :

An average NSE ëtait notë in 72 patients (72%). Seventeen patients (17%) had a low NSE, and 11 patients (11%) had an NSE ëкyë.

1.3.3. Educational level :

The ë educational level was university in 67.3% of patients, secondary in 23.5% and primary in 9.2%.

1.3.4. Habitat :

Eighty-two patients (82%) lived in urban areas and 18 (18%) in rural areas.

1.4. ANAMNESTIC CHARACTERISTICS :

1.4.1. Family history of celiac disease :

In our ëample, 35 patients (35%) had familial antëcëdents of CD.

1.4.2. Personal history of autoimmune diseases:

Of the patients with parйc1pë a l^tude, 24 (24%) had personal ATCD of autoimmune disease, with type 1 diabëte ë being the most common disease (10%).

The different personal antëcëdents of autoimmune disease in the population are rësumësed in Table I.

Table I: Personal history of autoimmune diseases in the study population :

	Frequency (n)	Percentage (%)
Personal history of autoimmune disease	24	24,0
Diabetes 10		10,0

Autoimmune hepatitis	5	2,0
Dysthyroidism 09		7,0

1.4.3. Lifestyle habits :

We identified 22 patients (22%) who were smokers and 78 patients (78%) who were non-smokers.

1.5. CLINICAL CHARACTERISTICS :

1.5.1. Age of onset of the disease :

The mëdian age of disease discovery in our population ëwas 11 years [IIQ= 2-30] with extremes ranging from 1 to 37 years. Fifty-four patients were younger than 20 years at the time of disease diagnosis.

1.5.2. Duration of the disease :

The median duration of CD was 21.5 years [IIQ= 6.25-28] with extremes ranging from 1 to 52 years.

1.6. EVALUATION OF RSG MEMBERSHIP:

Based on the Biagi score, 73 (73%) patients did not comply with a strict RSG (Figure 7).

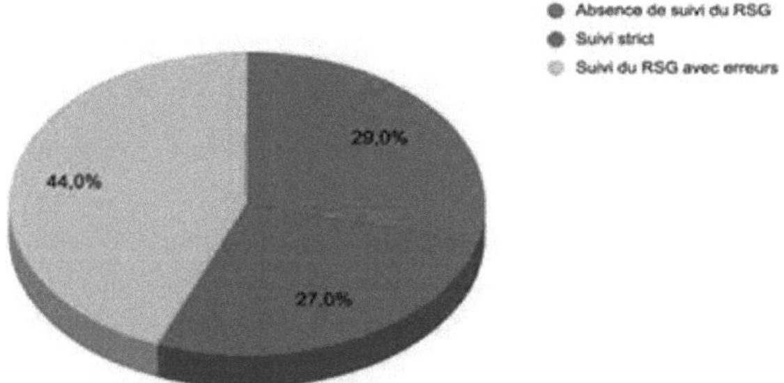

Figure 3: Distribution of patients according to adherence to the RSG according to the Biagi score

1.7. ASSESSMENT OF PATIENTS' quality of life:

1.7.1. Quality of life according to the SF12 questionnaire:

All patients in the sample had a global SF-12 score< 40 corresponding to an HRQ акёгёе. Physical HRQoL ё1.ай more акёгёе than mental HRQoL.

The mean scores for the physical and mental components and the overall mean score for the SF-12 are shown in Table II.

Table II: Patients' quality of life according to the SF12 questionnaire

	Mental component	Physical component	Total score
Average	14,33	12,00	26,00
Standard deviation	2,54	2,29	4,01
Minimum	6	7	13
Maximum	22	17	37

1.7.2. Quality of life according to the CDQ :

The CDQ domain related to ётойогс had the lowest mean (27.83 ± 7.65.

The mean scores for the four CDQ dimensions as well as the overall mean score are rësumës in Table III.

Table III: Patients' quality of life according to the CDQ questionnaire

	Emotions	Social problems	Inquiëtudes	Gastrointestinal symptoms	Total score
Average	27,83	31,38	29,32	33,43	123,86
Standard deviation	7,65	9,25	8,90		8,3029,57
Minimum	12,00	11,00	11,00	13,00	56,00
Maximum	46,00	49,00	49,00	49,00	181,00

2. ANALYTICAL STUDY: FACTORS ASSOCIATED WITH IMPAIRMENT OF QUALITY OF LIFE

2.1. UNIVARIATE ANALYSIS :

2.1.1. Study of the association between SF-12 and different variables

2.1.1.1. Patient-related variables:

Univariate analysis of factors associated with the SF-12 score showed that the physical component score was significantly lower in :

> Women compared with men (11.78±2.15 versus 12.89±2.47; p=0.02).

> Patients with a non-university education compared with those with a university education (11.00±1.93 versus 12.60±2.28; p=<0.001).

> Patients who had an autoimmune disease associated with their CD compared with those who did not (11.29±1.85 versus 12.34±2.36; p=0.004).

Non-university education was also associated with a lower total SF-12 score, the difference being statistically significant (p<0.001).

Table IV summarises the impact of different patient-related factors on QoL as assessed by the SF-12.

Table IV: Impact of patient-related factors on quality of life as assessed by the SF-12

	Mental component	P	Physical component	P	SF-12 total	P
Gender						
Men	14,79±3,45	0,26	12,89±2,47	**0,02**	27,68±5,44	0,05
Woman	15,15±2,08		11,78±2,15		25,93±3,35	
Age						
<40	14,57±2,63	0,13	12,22±2,49	0,35	26,79±4,24	0,14
>=40 years	13,71±2,20		11,75±1,62		25,46±3,56	
Marital status						
No tапë	14,43±2,55	0,66	11,86±2,39	0,25	26,29±4,11	0,71
Mапë	14,20±2,54		12,39±2,13		26,59±4,11	
Socioeconomic level						
Low	14,24±2,04	0,75	11,06±1,98	0,07	25,29±2,46	0,41
Medium and easyë	14,04±2,35		12,05±2,10		26,09±3,82	
Smoking						
Yes	14,77±2 ;26	0,36	11,94±2,18	0,21	26±14±3,99	0,21

No	14 ;21±2,61		12,64±2,61		27,41±4,38	
Level of education						
Non-university	13,81±2,21	0,15	11,00±1,93	**0,00**	24,81±3,13	**0,00**
University	14,59±2,66		12,60±2,28		27,19±4,29	
Habitat						
Urban	14,39±2,72	0,56	12,24±2,34	0,12	26,63±4,32	0,22
Rural	14,00±1,45		11,29±1,89		25,29±2,68	
Family history of celiac disease						
Yes	14,60±2,79	0,43	12,29±2,21	0,53	26,89±4,33	0,40
No	14,18±2,39		11,98±2,33		26,17±3,97	
Antëcëdents of autoimmune disease						
Yes	13,63±2,23	0,11	11,29±1,85	**0,04**	24,92±3,33	**0,03**
No	14,55±2,60		12,34±2,36		26,89±4,12	

2.1.1.2. *Disease-related variables:*

In our sërie, neither age at diagnosis nor disease progression time nor RSG adherence had a statistically significant association with HRQOL.

The impact of the variables linked to CD are detailed in table V.

Table V: Impact of CD-related factors on quality of life as assessed by the SF-12

		Mental component	P	Physical component	P	SF-12 total	P
Age at diagnosis							
	<20	14,59±2,70	0,26	12,24±2,62	0,47	26,83±4,42	0,27
	>=20	14,02±2,31		11,91±1,83		25,93±3,64	
Duration of the disease							
	<=5	14,59±2,75	0,58	12,18±2,03	0,83	26,77±4,08	0,64
	>5	14,26±2,48		12,06±2,36		26,32±4,11	
Biagi score							
Absence of of the GFD	follow-up	14,48±2,32	0,83	11,79±2,07	0,64	26,28±3,76	0,84
GFD tracking with error		14,16±2,75		12,11±2,32		26,27±4,33	
Strict monitoring		14,44±2,47		12,37±2,48		26,81±4,15	

2.1.2. Study of the association between CDQ and the various variables:

2.1.2.1. *Patient-related variables :*

> In patients with non-university education, the total CDQ score as well as the scores for all domains, with the exception of social probUms, ëwere statistically lower compared to patients with university education.

> The 'emotions' domain score was lower in patients with associated autoimmune diseases, the difference being statistically significant (28.86±7.90 versus 24.70±5.93; p=0.02).

> Patients with a low socio-economic level had the lowest scores in all domains, and the difference was statistically significant with the exception of the emotions domain.

Table VI summarises the impact of the various patient-related factors on the QOL assessed by the CDQ.

Table VI: Impact of patient-related factors on quality of life as assessed by the CDQ

	Emotions	P	Social problems	P	Concerns	P	Gastrointestinal symptoms	P	Total score	P
Gender										
Men	29,92±8,14	0,09	30,25±9,66	0,45	27,96±10,55	0,35	33,26±9,47	0,91	120,45±33,85	0,52
Woman	27,02±7,35		31,83±9,11		30,00±8,00		33,48±7,90		125,38±27,68	
Age										
<40	28,10±7,61	0,59	30,95±9,24	0,47	29,84±8,49	0,44	32,92±8,17	0,33	124,00±28,64	0,74
>=40	27,17±7,84		32,50±9,36		28,13±9,87		34,76±8,67		122,09±32,33	
Marital status										
No marie	27,16±7,55	0,33	30,32±9,41	0,21	31,19±7,54	0,08	33,40±8,48	0,97	124,31±29,03	0,89
Marie	28,67±7,78		32,69±8,97		27,65±9,75		33,45±8,17		123,41±30,49	
Socio-economic level										
Low	24,31±5,16	0,06	24,91±7,32	**0,01**	23,27±8,42	**0,01**	29,25±6,29	**0,04**	100,00±19,05	**0,01**
Medium and comfortable	28,09±7,82		31,88±9,22		29,95±8,39		33,80±8,27		125,26±29,42	
Smoking										
Yes	29,27±7,32	0,31	32,42±9,30	0,55	29,66±10,22	0,87	32,57±8,64	0,59	119,57±32,01	0,54
No	27,41±7,74		31,08±9,27		29,24±8,63		33,66±8,25		124,91±29,14	
Level of education										
No university	25,33±6,69	**0,01**	29,15±10,53	0,16	25,85±7,94	**0,03**	30,23±7,98	**0,00**	111,05±29,65	**0,02**
University	29,19±7,64		32,16±8,68		30,65±8,95		35,01±8,08		128,53±28,39	
Living environment										
Urban	27,56±7,47	0,40	31,59±9,11	0,47	29,15±8,62	0,70	33,23±8,10	0,60	122,57±28,89	0,38
Rural	29,31±8,82		29,50±10,12		30.30±11.37		34,41±9,59		131,88±36,05	
Family history of celiac disease										
Yes	27,96±7,93	0,90	31,26±8,25	0,92	27,69±7,52	0,25	33,63±7,55	0,85	120,70±26,06	0,52
No	27,76±7,5		31,45±9,83		30,18±9,49		33,31±8,73		125,46±31,3	

	Emotions	P	Social problems	P	Concerns	P	Gastrointestinal symptoms	P	Total score	P
	7								5	
Personal history of autoimmune disease (immune)										
Yes	24,70±5,93	**0,02**	30,04±9,92	0,44	26,66±9,20	0,14	31,12±8,41	0,11	116,58±29,18	0,24
No	28,86±7,90		31,79±9,06		30,15±8,71		34,19±8,18		126,14±29,59	

2.1.2.2. *Disease-related variables:*

No statistically significant association between CD-related variables and HRQoL ëevaluated by the CDQ was ëtë found.

The impact of these variables on QoL is detailed in Table VI.

Table VII: Impact of CD-related factors on quality of life as assessed by the CDQ

	Emotions	P	Social problems	P	Concerns	P	Gastrointestinal symptoms	P	Total score	P
Age at diagnosis										
<20	27,73±7,57	0,88	31,02±9,43	0,68	29,97±9,55	0,50	33,51±8,52	0,90	124,30±31,06	0,88
>=20	27,95±7,83		31,79±9,12		28,61±8,18		33,31±8,31		123,31±28,12	
Duration of the disease										
<=5	27,85±6,84	0,99	31,54±8,37	0,92	29,47±7,54	0,94	32,23±7,96	0,46	126,00±25,03	0,75
>59	27,83±7,85		31,33±9,55		29,28±9,14		33,76±8,42		123,28±30,85	
Biagi score										
Lack of GFD monitoring	28,25±7,16	0,94	31,15±9,22	0,84	29,04±9,95	0,88	34,13±8,78	0,75	124,65±30,43	0,97
GFD follow-up with errors	27,72±8,55		31,95±9,16		29,88±8,45		33,53±8,03		123,00±29,94	
Strict monitoring	27,57±6,80		30,64±9,73		28,71±8,89		32,46±8,42		124,47±29,60	

2.2. MULTIVARIATE ANALYSIS :

2.2.1. Independent factors influencing the QOL assessed by the SF12 :

At the end of the multivariate analysis, the only factor independently associated with a low physical HRQOL score was the level of non-university education (в=0.24; p=0.02). (p=0.21 ; p=0.03 andIC95%[0.10 - 3.59]) (Table VII)

Table VIII: Independent factors influencing HRQoL assessed by the SF-12

Physical quality of life Overall quality of life

Level of education	Beta	P	[95%IC]	Beta	P	[95%IC]
non-university	0,24	0,02	[0,13-2,09]	0,21	0,03	[0,10-3,59]

2.2.2. Independent factors influencing the QOL assessed by the CDQ :

At the end of the multivariate analysis, the NSE was statistically associated with alteration in the 'social problems' domain of the CDQ score (Beta=0.24; p=0.02 and IC95%[0.76 - 12.30]) as well as with alteration in overall HRQ (в=0.25; p=0.04 andIC95%[1.05 - 42.50]) (Table VIII).

Table IXIndependent factors influencing HRQoL assessed by CDQ

Quality of social life Overall quality of life

]\г1л7ря11 ^лг1л- vea.u sooo economique	Beta	P	[95%IC]	Beta	P	[95%IC]
	0,24	0,02	[0,76_12,30]	0,25	0,04	[1,05_42,50]

4 DISCUSSION

1. KEY RESULTS :

A cross-sectional a visëe analytic тепёе study was conducted over a 3-month period from October 2023 to December 2023 of known CD patients who were members of ATMC.

All data were collected using an online questionnaire. In the end, the study involved 100 patients included by convenience sampling.

The mean age of the population was 34.5 ± 9.5 years, with a sex ratio (male/female) of 0.39.

The QOL assessment was carried out using two questionnaires: a general questionnaire (the SF-12) and a specific questionnaire (the CDQ). This is the first nationwide study to assess the QOL of celiac patients.

According to the SF-12 and establishing a threshold of 40, all patients had an altered QOL, with a mean score of 26.00 ±4.01.

> In a univariate study, the factors associated with poorer quality of life were :

Female gender (p=0.02), non-university education (p<0.001), and history of associated autoimmune diseases (p=0.04).

> In the multivariate study, the only independent factor associated with an alteration in HRQOL was non-university education (Beta=0.21; p=0.03; 95% CI [0.10; 3.59]).

Assessment of QOL using the CDQ resulted in a mean score of 123.86 ±29.57.

> In a univariate study, the factors associated with impairment of HRQOL were :

Low SEN (p=0.01), non-university education (p= 0.02) and personal history of autoimmune diseases (p=0.02).

> In a multivariate study, only low NSE was independently associated with impaired QDV (Beta=0.25; p=0.04; 95% IC [1.05; 42.50]).

The discussion will be organised into five parts. The first part will focus on the definition and relevance of HRQOL assessment in chronic diseases, in this case CD. The second part will be devoted to the different means of assessing HRQOL during CD and their main results. The fourth part will focus on the factors associated with impairment of HRQoL. Finally, the strengths and limitations of this work will be highlighted.

2. DEFINITION AND BENEFITS OF QDV ASSESSMENT :

HRQOL has different meanings, reflecting the experience, knowledge and values of each individual. Many definitions have been proposed, but the WHO definition, most often cited in the literature, describes it as "an individual's perception of his or her position in life in the context of culture and his or her value system in relation to goals, expectations and standards" (24). This concept integrates in a complex way the person's physical health, psychological state, level of independence, social relationships, personal beliefs and relationships with the ëvënements in their environment (24).

This is different from QoL, where factors other than those relating to health come into play,

Health-related HRQoL is better suited to the field of medical evaluation and is an outcome indicator for assessing the consequences of a disease, the effect of medical care procedures, or the effect of prevention policies. This concept is defined as "the subjective perception of the impact of health status (illness and treatment) on physical, psychological and social functioning and well-being" (25).

The evaluation of health-related QoL is a health priority that makes it possible to understand the repercussions of a certain pathology on the patient's physical, social and mental health (26) . Indeed, by identifying the specific areas of patients' lives that are affected by the disease, QoL assessment can reveal unmet needs and guide the development of additional services and support, all with a view to improving patient care (27).

During the course of CD, patients' QoL may be impacted by different mechanisms. On the one hand, disease symptoms, whether gastrointestinal or extra-digestive, can lead to a dëtërioration of the QoL by limiting daily activities and affecting well-being дёпёral. In addition, nutritional deficiencies associated with CD can lead to chronic fatigue, muscle weakness and mood disorders, thus affecting physical and mental HRQoL.

In social terms, the strict dietary restrictions imposed by the disease can make social interaction extremely difficult. Patients may feel isolated or misunderstood because of their specific diet, which could have a negative impact on their emotional and social well-being.

In conclusion, the influence of CD on patients' QoL is multidimensional, affecting physical, mental and social well-being. Health professionals must therefore be aware of the impact of this disease and of the major interest of studying the QoL during CD (28).

3. MEANS OF ASSESSING QDV DURING MC AND THEIR MAIN RESULTS :

The HRQoL related to health is measured using QoL scales. However, the quantitative approach to a quaiitative concept is not always easy. A ëcheiie of QDV measurement must be constructed in compliance with a rigorous scientific procedure.

Numerous questionnaires concerning health-related QOL are available, some, known as generic, are used for various diseases, while others, known as spëcific, are specifically intended for patients with CD.

According to Burger et al., it would be preferable to combine the two types of instrument in order to properly support the concepts of health-related HRQoL in CD, which is what we have adopted in this work (29).

3.1. GENERAL QUESTIONNAIRES :

Among the general questionnaires, the two most frequently used are the MOS- SF (MedicalOutcomeStudy Short Form), in its long version (SF-36) **(Appendix V)** or shortened version (SF-12) and the HADS (Hospital Anxiety and DepressionScale). **(Appendix VI)**

3.1.1. SF-36 and SF-12 :

The SF-36 is one of the most frequently used scales in studies and surveys, thanks to its conciseness, high reproducibility, validity and sensitivity to change. In terms of QOL assessment, the SF-36 is currently considered the gold standard. It is used to establish a health and well-being profile based on 36 items divided into eight dimensions (physical activity, limitations due to physical condition, physical pain, general health, vitality, life and relationships with others, mental health and limitations due to psychological condition).

In order to have a simpler version of this questionnaire, Ware et al. developed an abbreviated form, the SF-12, comprising only 12 of the 36 questions, but covering the same dimensions and retaining the same validity (20). It has been used in major surveys of general and specific populations, and has been translated and validated in 141 languages.

Given its reliability, simplicity and availability in Arabic, we conducted our study using the SF-12. According to this score and establishing a threshold of 40, all the patients in our study had an altered HRQOL. Both the physical and mental components were affected.

The main advantage of using this type of general questionnaire is that it offers the possibility of comparing the QOL of patients with that of the general population. In making this comparison, we noted that the physical, mental and global HRQOL scores were all significantly lower than those of the general Tunisian population, with reference to the results of the validation study of the SF-12 in Tunisia (30).

Table IX compares the results of our study with those of the general Tunisian population.

Table X: Quality of life of patients as assessed by the SF-12 compared with the general population

	Component score	
	Physical	**mental**
General Tunisian population	50,14 ± 8,51	47,93± 9,85
Our sample	12,00±2,29	14,33±2,54

This alteration in HRQOL occasioned by CD has ële been confirmed by several ëtudes such as the study done by Tontini et al and that done by Lee et al (31,32) .

However, some studies have found no significant positive or negative impact of CD on QoL compared with the general population, such as the study by Cranney et al (33).

This disparity in results can be attributed, among other things, to the socio-cultural and economic differences between the study populations.

Table X summarises the results of the main studies assessing the impact of CD on health-related HRQoL using SF-12.

Table XI: Results of QoL assessment using the SF-12 in different studies

Authors	**Country**	**Year**	**Workforce**	**Score SF-12**	
				Physical component	**Mental component**
Cranney et al(33)	Canada	2007	2681	48	50
Tontini et al(31)	Italy	2010	43	49,10	42,30
Lee et al(32)	United States	2012	1743	38,12	36,79
C Deepak et al(34)	India	2018	60	37,20	41,88
Our study	Tunisia	2024	100	12,00	14,33

3.1.2. The HADS questionnaire :

The HADS is a specially designed questionnaire for assessing anxiety and depression in patients with physical illnesses. It comprises two domains from which two scores can be calculated. If one of the latter 2 is >11, this could be indicative of a probable mental disorder (35).

This questionnaire was used by Hauser et al in their study carried out in 2006, which concluded that creeliac patients had a reduced HRQoL compared with the general population (36).

3.2. SPECIFIC QUESTIONNAIRES :

Generic questionnaires may not adequately capture the attitudes, perceptions and needs that are spëcifically related to CD and this may lead to less sensitive results hence the need to use spëcific means to achieve more accurate and valid results.

Several questionnaires to assess QOL have been designed specifically for patients with CD, the most widely used being the CDQ and the CeliacDiseaseQuality Of Lifesurvey (CD-QOL)

(22,37).

3.2.1. CDQ :

The CDQ is a relatively recent instrument that was first developed in a German version in 2007 by Hauser et al (22). The domains were constructed by factor analysis to address clinical criteria such as bowel symptoms, psychological well-being and social functioning, while being comparable to domains used in questionnaires for other gastrointestinal diseases such as inflammatory bowel disease (38).

A list of items was initially selected from the literature and from other questionnaires used to assess HRQoL in celiac patients such as the BI (Burden of Illness), SAIC (Self-Administered Inventory for Celiacs), questions on social restrictions specific to CD from a Canadian survey and other studies that have explored the welfare issues associated with CD(39,40). Some items were also based on the IBDQ (InflammatoryBowelDisease Questionnaire) in order to assess the emotional and social well-being of celiac patients. Finally, appropriate questions were constructed for each item with 7 possible response options based on a Likert scale.

The CDQ has been translated into several languages and has been validated in several countries, including Italy, Spain, France, Turkey, Brazil, Iran, Argentina, Portugal and recently Morocco (23, 41-48).

This questionnaire has ële subsequently adoptedë for re-evaluation of the QDV of celiacs in several ëtudies, which have shown total scores far from the maximum score (196), some of which are comparable to the results of our ëtude(44-47).

Table XI summarises the results of the main ëstudies that have ëvaluatedë the impact of CD on QDV Hëc a la sante by means of CDQ.

Table XII: CDQ quality of life assessment results from different studies

Author	Country	Year	Workforce	Total CDQ score
Hauser et al(22)	Germany	2007	488	151
Chaves et al(49)	Portugal	2013	234	103,28
A. Marchese et al(41)	Italy	2013	171	159
C. P. Pratesi et al(45)	Brazil	2018	450	119
Aksan et al(44)	Turkey	2015	205	124
F. Barzegar et al(46)	Iran	2018	81	119
Selleski et al(47)	Argentina	2020	171	124
Harnett and Myers(50)	Australia	2020	45	147
Our study	Tunisia	2023	100	123

3.2.2. CD-QOL :

The CD-QOL was developed by Dorn et al. in 2010 (37). **(Appendix VII)**

This is a specific and valid instrument for assessing quality of life in CD, comprising 20 questions divided into four areas: limitations, dysphoria, health problems and inadequate treatment. The questions were developed after gathering information relating to the nature of the disease and its impact on daily life from focus groups of patients with CD. The questions were then studied by experts to produce a preliminary version of the questionnaire.

The latter was administered in turn to other patients and finally a validation study was ëtë тепëe to ë assess the psychomotor propriës of this questionnaire.

The CD-QOL was ëtë uh^rieurely translated into Italian in 2012 and Spanish in 2013 (42.51) and has

ëtë usedë in several ëtudes which led to its psychomëtric validation(52-55).

Unlike the CDQ, the CD-QOL does not include items relating to the physical impact of CD, as patients in the Dorn study did not report these as major concerns.

It should be noted that these two specific questionnaires were not formally compared.

3.2.3. Other specific questionnaires :

There are other specific questionnaires for CD, but they are less commonly used than the CDQ or CD-QOL, such as the CCHS (Canadian Celiac Health Survey) developed by Cranney et al in 2007 and comprising 76 questions, and the BI (Burden of Illness) developed by Swedish authors and comprising 9 items(33,39) .

4. FACTORS INFLUENCING QDV IN MC :

4.1. PATIENT-RELATED FACTORS :

4.1.1. Genre:

The effect of gender on HRQoL during CD has been ëtë ëvaluatedë by several ëtudies, and fëminor sex has ëtë foundë to be a factor significantly associated with higher HRQoL. Thus, in the Argentine study by Selleski et al, women had the lowest scores compared with men in all domains, with a statistically significant difference (p=0.006) (47). These results were also found in the study by Moreno et al and Pratesi et al (45,56).

Several hypotheses for these results are frequently reported in ëtudes. Indeed, psychosocial factors may play a greater role in women than in men. In addition, women have greater concerns and worëtudes related to the disease and its impact on body image. The fact that this finding is also found in the majority of studies conducted in general populations further supports these hypotheses.

In our study, physical HRQOL was significantly worse in women than in men (11.78±2.15 versus 12.89±2.47; p=0.02). According to these hypotheses, this difference would therefore be unrelated to the impact of CD on HRQOL. Especially since, based on the CDQ, no significant association was found between gender and HRQoL. These results corroborate those of studies by Aksan et al and Pouchot et alou, who found no significant differences in the overall CDQ score and its domains between the two sexes (43,44).

4.1.2. Age :

In our study, age was not associated with impairment of HRQOL, whether assessed by the general or specific questionnaire. This same result was reported in the Portuguese study, the Argentinean study and the Turkish study (44,47,49).

However, some authors have highlighted the influence of age on the HRQ of celiac patients. Moreno et al. indicated that age was inversely associated with the different domains of the CDQ (56). This finding, also found in the general population, is not directly related to CD, but rather to the increased incidence of associated comorbidities and to age-related morbidity.

Marital status :

Few studies have examined the association between HRQOL and marital status. In our series, no statistically significant association was found. This is in line with the results of the Portuguese study and those of a Slovenian cohort of 247 patients. It should be noted that, in these studies as well as our own, the scores were slightly higher in married patients, which could be explained by the role of the family in providing support and help in coping with the disease.

4.1.3. Educational level:

Our study showed a significant association of the non-university educational level with the alteration of the QDV with both the general and the specific questionnaires. This factor also emerged as a factor indĕpendant Hë a l'ah^ration de la QDV avec le SF-12 dans la composante physique et dans le score total.

This significant association between HRQOL and educational level has been reported in several other studies, such as the Brazilian study by Pratesi et al, where a significant association between a high level of education and good HRQOL was noted(45).

These results could be explained by the fact that patients with a high level of education are better informed, have a better understanding of their disease, and are consequently less anxious than patients with a secondary or primary level of education(57).

On the other hand, the Portuguese study by Chaves et al on 234 celiac patients showed that the higher the level of education, the poorer the quality of life (49). The hypothesis that could explain this finding suggests that patients with a low level of education would be less socially active, and would be less preoccupied by their state of health, which would have less of an impact on quality of life.

4.1.4. Socio-economic level:

In our series, low NSE ëwas an indĕpendant Kë factor in HRQOL impairment. This finding is in agreement with those of most studies found in the literature that report a significant association between HRQOL and NSE. In the study by Zysk et al. published in 2018, which included 251 patients, patients with a poorer economic situation had significantly lower scores on the emotional, social and "worries" subscales of the CDQ compared with patients reporting a better economic situation (15).

Similarly, a retrospective cohort study by Roy et al in 2016 found that income modulates both health care seeking and access to health care facilities, implying that patients from a low socio-economic class would be less likely to be diagnosed and treated, resulting in impaired quality of life (58).

4.1.5. Habitat :

Several studies have shown a significant impact of the living environment on patients' quality of life. In the Moroccan study by M. *Guennounet al*, a statistically significant association was found between the living environment and all domains of the CDQ(23) .

Indeed, those living in urban areas had higher scores than those living in rural areas. The authors suggested that this could be explained mainly by the difficulties encountered by patients living in rural areas in accessing healthcare facilities.

However, in our series, we did not find an association between living environment and HRQoL, and this may be due to the low percentage of patients living in rural areas in our sample (18%).

4.1.6. Smoking :

The study of the QOL of Spanish adults carried out by Moreno et al in 2022 showed a statistically significant association between smoking and QOL, with non-smokers having higher scores in the areas of emotions and gastrointestinal symptoms (56) .

However, in our work we did not find a statistically significant association between smoking status and HRQoL. The discrepancy in the results between the two series can be explained mainly by the specificity of the sample studied in the survey carried out by Moreno et al.

4.1.7. History of associated autoimmune diseases:

In our study, in univariate analysis, patients with no personal history of autoimmune disease had the highest scores on either the SF-12 or the CDQ. However, after adjustment, this factor did not appear to be an independent factor.

This is in line with the results of the Slovenian study cited above, in which dysthyroidism and diabetes were reported as factors influencing HRQoL, but were not retained as independent factors by the logistic regression method.

In contrast, Paarlahti et al showed, in a large cross-sectional study of 596 patients, that dysthyroidism was a factor independently associated with impaired HRQoL (OR= 2.02; 95%CI[1.29-3.16]; p=0.002)(59). In fact, untreated dysthyroidism is associated with gastrointestinal symptoms which generally disappear with treatment (60).

In reality, the specific interaction between other associated autoimmune diseases and their influence on QoL has rarely been the subject of in-depth analysis. That said, it is legitimate to consider that the presence of comorbidities may contribute to a higher burden of CD.

4.2. FACTORS LINKED TO THE DISEASE :

4.2.1. Development time :

The results of studies in the literature on the influence of the duration of illness on HRQOL are contradictory.

Indeed, Zysk et al showed that the time taken for the disease to progress had no impact on HRQoL(15). The same was true of the Argentinian study, which found no association between the time taken to diagnose CD and HRQOL(47). These results were consistent with our own.

In contrast, a cross-sectional study conducted in two tertiary referral centres in Mexico showed that CD patients with a longer duration of progression had a better quality of life (61). This could be explained by the fact that a long course of the disease gives the patient time to adapt, to live better with the disease and its symptoms, and indicates better adaptation in relation to the restrictions imposed by the GSR. The idea of adaptation to the GFD over the years was well supported by the study carried out in southern Brazil by A. C. *Castilhos* et *al*, in which newly-diagnosed patients (< 1 year) were compared with those whose disease had progressed over a longer period (> 10 years) (62). The latter actually had a better quality of life.

4.2.2. Age at diagnosis

As with the duration of the disease, the results on the impact of age at diagnosis are also divergent. On the one hand, Hauser et al. found that a younger age at diagnosis induced a poorer quality of life, as did Ciacci et al(40,63) . The hypothesis put forward by the authors is that psychological adaptation to CD and GTR is more difficult for children and adolescents than for adults. Thus, it could be that adolescents with adjustment problems remain more confronted with these problems in adulthood than those diagnosed later in life.

On the other hand, the Portuguese study by C. Chaves et al concluded that the younger the age at diagnosis (less than 20 years), the better the HRQoL(49). This may be due to difficulties in accepting the GPR when the diagnosis is made at a later age.

However, in our series and that of the Argentine study, no significant association was demonstrated (47).

4.2.3. Membership of the RSG :

The effect of adherence to the GFD on the quality of life of celiacs is a controversial subject. Indeed, some studies have demonstrated a positive impact of adherence to the GFD, such as the study conducted by Johnston et al, which found a significant improvement after 1 year of GFD(64). Scandinavian studies have also shown that the quality of life of celiac patients strictly adherent to the GFD for 10 years with histological and serological remission was comparable to that of the general population (65,66).

Similarly, in the series by Hauser et al. there was a significant association between non-adherence to the GSR and reduced HRQOL(63). However, this conclusion should be qualified, given that the evaluation of adherence to the GSR was based on self-assessment, which is subjective by definition.

In this study, in order to objectively assess adherence to the RSG, we used a valid score: the Biagi score. It is interesting to note that, according to this score, only 27% of our sample adhered to a strict RSG. This low percentage could be explained essentially by the high cost and lack of availability and variety of gluten-free products, making the GFD a real economic burden. The lack of reimbursement by the national health insurance fund also contributes to this burden. This issue has also been raisedëe in other countries such as Morocco where the cost and availability^ of gluten-free products constituted a bвтёге to good adherence to the regime (67). This was also highlighted in the Iranian cohort where patients faced burdensome expenses that were unaffordable for many of them (68).

Given скпё the importance of GFD compliance for disease control and the avoidance of complications, as well as the potential impact on QoL, some countries have implemented measures to help and support patients. In France, partial reimbursement of gluten-free products was introduced in 2004 (69). In the UK, as in several other Anglo-Saxon countries, a number of gluten-free foods can be obtained free of charge on prescription(70,71).

When we compared the HRQoL of strict adherents and non-adherents or partial adherents to the RSG, we did not dëmontrë any significant difference. This is consistent with the results of M. Guennouni et al, A. Marchese et al and Zysk et al (15,23,41) . The lack of impact of adherence to the GFD on QoL could be explained by the fact that the beneficial effects of the regimen may be counterbalanced by the constraints it imposes on patients. In addition to the economic constraints described above, the diet can impose a considerable mental burden on various aspects of daily life.

This overload is the result of efforts to avoid gluten, which can lead to feelings of frustration and deprivation. In fact, this overload appears to be greatest at the beginning of the diet, when people are learning which products are allowed and which are to be eliminated, which can require a considerable investment of time and energy.

5. STRENGTHS AND LIMITATIONS OF THE STUDY :

5.1. HIGHLIGHTS OF OUR STUDY :

^   To our knowledge, our study constitutes the first study in Tunisia to intëresse the QOL of celiac patients with an objective ëvaluation using both a general questionnaire (SF-12) and a specific questionnaire (CDQ).

^   The choice of target population (members of the ATMC) and the use of an online questionnaire enabled the study to be disseminated more widely without the participants being directly confronted by the investigator. This reduced the discomfort associated especially with the evaluation of the follow-up of the RSG and its violations, leading to more accurate results on adherence to the regime and on QoL in a general manière.

^ Adherence to the RSG was assessed using a valid score (the Biagi), providing reliable results and an objective assessment.

5.2. LIMITATIONS OF THE STUDY :

^ The main limitation of our study was the type of sampling used: non-probabilistic convenience sampling, which could create a selection bias. Nevertheless, we applied it in order to achieve a larger sample size and to recruit patients from all regions of the country.

^ Patients who are members of the ATMC are aware of the issue of CD; non-members could not be included. This is therefore a population with special characteristics compared with the real population.

^ The cross-sectional nature of the study makes it impossible to establish the temporal sequence of the evènements and implies a reservation in ^causal interpretation of the associations found.

6. RECOMMENDATIONS :

❖ It would be reasonable to generalise the assessment of QOL in patients with CD, particularly those with factors predictive of poorer QOL (female gender, low NSE, non-university educational level, autoimmune disease, etc.).

Immuneassociee), during their outpatient follow-up. This ëassessment would make it possible to:

^ To assess the impact of celiac disease on the daily lives of sufferers

^ Track revolution and the impact of the disease over time and include a longitudinal perspective.

^ Dëcisëment of the aspects of life affected by the disease and the challenges faced by patients on a daily basis so that effective action can be taken and care improved, in this case by offering psychological support where necessary.

^ Strengthen the doctor-patient relationship by communicating to the practitioner the issues and problems that patients face on a daily basis and receiving psychological support in return.

❖ It could also be beneficial to involve family and friends in care, given the significant social impact of this disease in terms of limiting socialisation and relationships because of GMS. With this in mind, we need to :

^ Start by providing psychological counselling for patients.

^ Organise consultations with the patient's family and friends to raise their awareness of their role in the overall care of the patient, stressing the importance of the psychological support they can provide.

^ Educate the patient's family and friends about the disease as a whole, and specifically about the GMSR, to help the patient adapt to it and accept it less painfully, so that they are more likely to adhere to it.

❖ It is also important to raise awareness among health authorities in order to facilitate access to care and contribute to the reimbursement of gluten-free foods and products, which are often more expensive than their gluten-containing equivalents. This would make it possible to reduce the financial burden associated with GFD and guarantee a better quality of life for people suffering from this disease.

5 CONCLUSION

CD is an autoimmune disorder whose incidence is constantly increasing. It is distinguished, on the one hand, by its great clinical polymorphism, and on the other, by the particularity of its therapeutic management, which remains mainly diëtetic, axëe on a strict lifelong GFD. The influence of CD on patients' QoL is multidimensional, involving its symptoms, the nutritional deficiencies it induces, and ëgalement the constraints presented by adherence to the RSG. Thus, healthcare professionals must be aware of the impact of this disease and of the major importance of reassessing the quality of life of patients suffering from it.

It was with this in mind that we carried out this study, the aims of which were to assess the impact of CD on patients' quality of life and to identify the factors that might influence it.

To this end, we conducted a descriptive and analytical cross-sectional study over a three-month period from 1er October to 31 December 2023, which included 100 patients who were members of the ATMC. We used two valid tools for evaluating QoL, available in Arabic: a general questionnaire (the SF-12) and a questionnaire specific to CD (the CDQ).

Our population was predominantly female, with a sex ratio (male/female) of 0.39. The mean age was 34.5 ± 9.5 years. Half of the patients were single at the time of the questionnaire. The SEN was mostly average (72%), low in 17% of cases, and comfortable in 11% of the population. The level of education was university in 67.3% of patients. Patients living in urban areas represented 82% of the study population. Active smoking was recorded in 22% of patients.

In our sample, 35% of patients had a family history of CD and 24% had a personal history of an autoimmune disease associated with CD, with type 1 diabetes being the most common (10%).

The median age at onset of the disease in our population was 11 years [IIQ= 2-30] with a median duration of 21.5 years [IIQ= 6.25-28].

With regard to adherence to the GFD, based on a validated score (the Biagi score), it was noted that the majority of patients followed the regimen with errors (44%). Only 27% of patients adhered to a strict RSG.

The mean SF-12 total score was 26.00 ± 4.01. The mean scores for the mental and physical components were 14.33 ± 2.54 and 12.00 ± 2.29 respectively. All patients had scores below 40, corresponding to altered HRQOL.

The spëcific evaluation by the CDQ objective a mean global score of 123.86 ± 29.57 out of a maximum score of 196. The gastrointestinal symptoms domain had the highest mean (33.43 ± 8.00) and the emotions domain had the lowest mean (27.83 ± 7.65).

The analytical part of our ëtude concerned the identification of factors associated with the deterioration of patients' QOL.

Based on SF-12:

> In a univariate study, the factors associated with poorer quality of life were :

> Female gender (p=0.02), non-university education (p<0.001), and history of associated autoimmune diseases (p=0.04).

> In the multivariate study, the only independent factor associated with an alteration in HRQOL was non-university education (Beta=0.21; p=0.03; 95% CI [0.10; 3.59]).

According to the CDQ :

> In a univariate study, the factors associated with impairment of HRQOL were :

Low SEN (p=0.01), non-university education (p= 0.02) and personal history of autoimmune diseases (p=0.02).

> In a multivariate study, only low NSE was independently associated with impaired QDV (Beta=0.25; p=0.04; 95% IC [1.05; 42.50]).

In summary, our study proves that CD alters the QOL of Tunisian patients. It has enabled us to identify the factors associated with this alteration in QOL.

Our results suggest that the use of QOL assessment tools should be generalised, particularly specific tools such as the CDQ. This would open up prospects for psvchotherapeutic intervention in patients with CD aimed at optimising their management. Furthermore, our ёstudy highlights the interest and need to implement assistance and support strategies for celiac patients, in order to reduce the burden of the disease and improve adherence to the GFD, which remains the main guarantor of a favourable ёvolution without complications.

6 REFERENCES

1. Vauquelin B, Riviere P. Celiac disease. La Revue de Mĕdecme Interne. 1 oct2023;44(10):539-45.

2. Lebwohl B, Rubio-Tapia A. Epidemiology, Presentation, and Diagnosis of CeliacDisease. Gastroenterology. Jan 2021;160(1):63-75.

3. Catassi C, Verdu EF, Bai JC, Lionetti E. Coeliacdisease. The Lancet. 25 June 2022;399(10344):2413-26.

4. Bdioui F, Sakly N, Hassine M, Saffar H. Prevalence of celiac disease in Tunisian blood donors. Chistroenterologie Clinique et Biologique. Jan 2006;30(1):33-6.

5. Gargouri L, Kolsi N, Maalej B, Weli M, Mahfoudh A. MALADIE CCILIAQUL CHEZ L'ENFANT CELIAC DISEASE IN CHILDREN.

6. Costa S, Astarita L, Ben-Hariz M, Curro G, Dolinsek J, Kansu A, et al. A Point-of-Care test for facing the burden of undiagnosed celiac disease in the Mediterranean area: a pragmatic design study. BMC Gastroenterol. dĕc 2014;14(1):219.

7. Caio G, Volta U, Sapone A, Leffler DA, De Giorgio R, Catassi C, et al. Celiac disease: a comprehensive current review. BMC Med. dĕc 2019;17(1):142.

8. van Gils T, Rootsaert B, Bouma G, Mulder CJJ. Celiac Disease in The Netherlands: Demographic Data of Members of the Dutch Celiac Society. J GastrointestinLiver Dis. dĕc 2016;25(4):441-5.

9. celiac-disease-english-2016.pdf [Internet]. [cйё 7 May 2024]. Available from: https://www.worldgastroenterology.org/UserFiles/file/guidelines/celiac-disease-french-2016.pdf

10. Chand N, Mihas AA. Celiac Disease: Current Concepts in Diagnosis and Treatment. Journal of Clinical Gastroenterology. Jan 2006;40(1):3.

11. Meyer D, Shane E. Osteoporosis in a North American Adult Population With Celiac Disease. 2001;96(1).

12. Cosnes J, Nion-Larmurier I. Complications of celiac disease. PathologieBiologie. 1 Apr 2013;61(2):e21-6.

13. Green PHR, Fleischauer AT, Bhagat G, Goyal R, Jabri B, Neugut AI. Risk of malignancy in patients with celiac disease. Am J Med. 15 August 2003;115(3):191-5.

14. Guennouni M, Elkhoudri N, Bourrhouat A, Hilali A. Assessment of quality of life in children, adolescents, and adults with celiac disease through specific questionnaires: Review. Clinical Nutrition and Mĕtabolism. 1 Oct 2020;34(3):194-200.

15. Zysk W, Glqbska D, Guzek D. Social and Emotional Fears and Worries Influencing the Quality of Life of Female Celiac Disease Patients Following a Gluten-Free Diet. Nutrients. Oct 2018;10(10):1414.

16. Fera T, Cascio B, Angelini G, Martini S, Guidetti CS. Affective disorders and quality of life in adult coeliac disease patients on a gluten-free diet. Eur J Gastroenterol Hepatol. dĕc 2003;15(12):1287-92.

17. Biagi F, Andrealli A, Bianchi PI, Marchese A, Klersy C, Corazza GR. A gluten-free diet score to evaluate dietary compliance in patients with coeliac disease. Br J Nutr. 28 Sep 2009;102(6):882-7.

18. Biagi F, Bianchi PI, Marchese A, Trotta L, Vattiato C, Balduzzi D, et al. A score that verifies adherence to a gluten-free diet: a cross-sectional, multicentre validation in real clinical life. Br J Nutr. 28 Nov 2012;108(10):1884-8.

19. Ware J, Kosinski M, Gandek B. SF-36 Health Survey: Manual & Interpretation Guide. Lincoln, RI: QualityMetric Incorporated. 1 Jan 1993;

20. Ware JE, Kosinski M, Keller SD. A 12-Item Short-Form Health Survey: Construction of Scales and Preliminary Tests of Reliability and Validity. Medical Care. March 1996;34(3):220.

21. Haddad C, Sacre H, Obeid S, Salameh P, Hallit S. Validation of the Arabic version of the "12-item short-form health survey" (SF-12) in a sample of Lebanese adults. Arch Public Health. dec 2021;79(1):56.

22. Hauser W, Gold J, Stallmach A, Caspary WF, Stein J. Development and Validation of the Celiac Disease Questionnaire (CDQ), a Disease-specific Health-related Quality of Life Measure for Adult Patients With Celiac Disease. Journal of Clinical Gastroenterology. Feb 2007;41(2):157-66.

23. Guennouni M, Admou B, Elkhoudri N, Bouchrit S, Ait Rami A, Bourrahouat A, et al. Quality of life of Moroccan patients with celiac disease: Arabic translation, cross-cultural adaptation, and validation of the celiac disease questionnaire. Arab J Gastroenterol. Nov 2022;23(4):246-52.

24. Study protocol for the World Health Organization project to develop a Quality of Life assessment instrument (WHOQOL). Qual Life Res. Apr 1993;2(2):153-9.

25. Bradley C. Importance of differentiating health status from quality of life. Lancet. 6 Jan 2001;357(9249):7-8.

26. Eisen GM, Locke RGI, Provenzale D. Health-Related Quality of Life: A Primer for Gastroenterologists. Official journal of the American College of Gastroenterology | ACG. August 1999;94(8):2017.

27. Ninot G. Health-related quality of life in chronic diseases. In:Bacro F, ëditeur. La qualite de vie: Approches psychologiques [Internet]. Rennes: Presses universitaires de Rennes; 2014 [cited 13 Feb 2024]. p. 117-37. (Psychologies). Available from: https://books.openedition.org/pur/61283

28. Zingone F, Swift GL, Card TR, Sanders DS, Ludvigsson JF, Bai JC. Psychological morbidity of celiac disease: A review of the literature. United European Gastroenterology Journal. 2015;3(2):136-45.

29. Burger JPW, Van Middendorp H, Drenth JPH, Wahab PJ, Evers AWM. How to best measure quality of life in coeliac disease? A validation and comparison of diseasespecific and generic quality of life measures. European Journal of Gastroenterology & Hepatology. August 2019;31(8):941-7.

30. Younsi M. Health-Related Quality-of-Life Measures: Evidence from Tunisian Population Using the SF-12 Health Survey. Value in Health Regional Issues. Sept 2015;7:54-66.

31. Tontini GE, Rondonotti E, Saladino V, Saibeni S, De Franchis R, Vecchi M. Impact of Gluten Withdrawal on Health-Related Quality of Life in Celiac Subjects: An Observational Case-Control Study. Digestion. 2010;82(4):221-8.

32. Lee AR, Ng DL, Diamond B, Ciaccio EJ, Green PHR. Living with coeliac disease: survey results from the U.S.A. J Hum Nutr Diet. June 2012;25(3):233-8.

33. Cranney A, Zarkadas M, Graham ID, Butzner JD, Rashid M, Warren R, et al. The Canadian Celiac Health Survey. Dig Dis Sci. March 21, 2007;52(4):1087-95.

34. C D, Berry N, Vaiphei K, Dhaka N, Sinha SK, Kochhar R. Quality of life in celiac disease and the effect of gluten-free diet. JGH Open. 2018;2(4):124-8.

35. Zigmond AS, Snaith RP. The Hospital Anxiety and Depression Scale. Acta Psychiatr

Scand. June 1983;67(6):361-70.

36. H??user W, Gold J, Stein J, Caspary WF, Stallmach A. Health-related quality of life in adult coeliac disease in Germany: results of a national survey: European Journal of Gastroenterology & Hepatology. juill 2006;18(7):747-54.

37. Dorn SD, Hernandez L, Minaya MT, Morris CB, Hu Y, Leserman J, et al. The development and validation of a new coeliac disease quality of life survey (CD-QOL). Alimentary Pharmacology & Therapeutics. March 2010;31(6):666-75.

38. Guyatt G, Mitchell A, Irvine EJ, Singer J, Williams N, Goodacre R, et al. A new measure of health status for clinical trials in inflammatory bowel disease. Gastroenterology. March 1989;96(3):804-10.

39. Hallert C, Granno C, I lulten S, Midhagen G, Strom M, Svensson H, et al. Living with coeliac disease: controlled study of the burden of illness. Scand J Gastroenterol. Jan 2002;37(1):39-42.

40. Ciacci C, Iavarone A, Siniscalchi M, Romano R, De Rosa A. Psychological dimensions of celiac disease: toward an integrated approach. Dig Dis Sci. Sept 2002;47(9):2082-7.

41. Marchese A, Klersy C, Biagi F, Balduzzi D, Bianchi PI, Trotta L, et al. Quality of life in coeliac patients: Italian validation of a coeliac questionnaire. Eur J Intern Med. Jan 2013;24(1):87-91.

42. Casellas F, Rodrigo L, Molina-Infante J, Vivas S, Lucendo AJ, Rosinach M, et al. Transcultural adaptation and validation of the Celiac Disease Quality of Life (CD-QOL) Survey, a specific questionnaire to measure quality of life in patients with celiac disease. Rev EspEnferm Dig. 2013;105(10):585-93.

43. Pouchot J, Despujol C, Malamut G, Ecosse E, Coste J, Cellier C. Validation of a French Version of the Quality of Life "Celiac Disease Questionnaire". Assassi S, éditeur. PLoS ONE. 2 May 2014;9(5):e96346.

44. Aksan A, Mercanligil SM, Hauser W, Karaismailoglu E. Validation of the Turkish version of the Celiac Disease Questionnaire (CDQ). Health Qual Life Outcomes. 19 June2015;13:82.

45. Pratesi CP, Hauser W, Uenishi RH, Selleski N, Nakano EY, Gandolfi L, et al. Quality of Life of Celiac Patients in Brazil: Questionnaire Translation, Cultural Adaptation and Validation. Nutrients. 25 Aug 2018;10(9):1167.

46. Barzegar F, Pourhoseingholi MA, Rostami-Nejad M, Gholizadeh S, Malekpour MR, Sadeghi A, et al. Transcultural Adaptation and Validation of Persian Version of Celiac Disease Questionnaire (CDQ); A Specific Questionnaire to Measure Quality of Life of Iranian Patients. Galen Med J. 2018;7:e1106.

47. Selleski N, Zandonadi RP, Milde LB, Gandolfi L, Pratesi R, Hauser W, et al. Evaluation of Quality of Life of Adult Patients with Celiac Disease in Argentina: From Questionnaire Validation to Assessment. Int J Environ Res Public Health. 26 Sep 2020;17(19):7051.

48. Lobao C, Goncalves R, Monteiro BR. Desenvolvimento da versaoportuguesa do celiac disease questionnaire. SOCIAL REVIEW International Social Sciences Review / RevistaInternacional de CienciasSociales [Internet]. 6 March 2013 [сИё 15 fèvr 2024];2(1). Available from: https://journals.eagora.org/revSOCIAL/article/view/1229

49. Chaves C, Raposo A, Zandonadi RP, Nakano EY, Ramos F, Teixeira-Lemos E. Quality of Life Perception among Portuguese Celiac Patients: A Cross-Sectional Study Using the Celiac Disease Questionnaire (CDQ). Nutrients. 24 Apr 2023;15(9):2051.

50. Harnett JE, Myers SP. Quality of life in people with ongoing symptoms of coeliac disease

despite adherence to a strict gluten-free diet. Sci Rep. 24 Jan 2020;10(1):1144.

51. Zingone F, Iavarone A, Tortora R, Imperatore N, Pellegrini L, Russo T, et al. The Italian translation of the celiac disease-specific quality of life scale in celiac patients on gluten free diet. DigLiver Dis. fěvr 2013;45(2):115-8.

52. Casellas F, Rodrigo L, Lucendo AJ, Fernandez-Banares F, Molina-Infante J, Vivas S, et al. Benefit on health-related quality of life of adherence to gluten-free diet in adult patients with celiac disease. Rev EspEnferm Dig. Apr 2015;107(4):196-201.

53. Lee AR, Wolf R, Contento I, Verdeli H, Green PHR. Coeliac disease: the association between quality of life and social support network participation. J Hum Nutr Diet. June 2016;29(3):383-90.

54. Mahadev S, Gardner R, Lewis SK, Lebwohl B, Green PH. Quality of Life in Screen-detected Celiac Disease Patients in the United States. J Clin Gastroenterol. 2016;50(5):393-7.

55. Tennyson CA, Simpson S, Lebwohl B, Lewis S, Green PHR. Interest in medical therapy for celiac disease. Therap Adv Gastroenterol. Sep 1, 2013;6(5):358-64.

56. Moreno MDL, Sanchez-Munoz D, Sousa C. Quality of Life in Teenagers and Adults With Coeliac Disease: From Newly Spanish Coeliac Disease Questionnaire Validation to Assessment in a Population-Based Study. Front Nutr. May 31, 2022;9:887573.

57. Gazmararian JA, Williams MV, Peel J, Baker DW. Health literacy and knowledge of chronic disease. Patient Educ Couns. Nov 2003;51(3):267-75.

58. Roy A, Mehra S, Kelly CP, Tariq S, Pallav K, Dennis M, et al. The association between socioeconomic status and the symptoms at diagnosis of celiac disease: a retrospective cohort study. Therap Adv Gastroenterol. 1 Jul 2016;9(4):495-502.

59. Paarlahti P, Kurppa K, Ukkola A, Collin P, Huhtala H, Maki M, et al. Predictors of persistent symptoms and reduced quality of life in treated coeliac disease patients: a large cross-sectional study. BMC Gastroenterol. děc 2013;13(1):75.

60. Ebert EC. The thyroid and the gut. J Clin Gastroenterol. July 2010;44(6):402-6.

61. Ramfrez-Cervantes KL, Remes-Troche JM, del Pilar Milke-Garda M, Romero V, Uscanga LF. Characteristics and factors related to quality of life in Mexican Mestizo patients with celiac disease. BMC Gastroenterology. 22 Jan 2015;15(1):4.

62. Castilhos AC, Goncalves BC, Macedo E Silva M, Lanzoni LA, Metzger LR, Kotze LMS, et al. QUALITY OF LIFE EVALUATION IN CELIAC PATIENTS FROM SOUTHERN BRAZIL. Arq Gastroenterol. Sep 2015;52(3):171-5.

63. Hauser W, Stallmach A, Caspary WF, Stein J. Predictors of reduced health-related quality of life in adults with coeliac disease. Aliment PharmacolTher. March 2007;25(5):569-78.

64. Johnston SD, Rodgers C, Watson RGp. Quality of life in screen-detected and typical coeliac disease and the effect of excluding dietary gluten: European Journal of Gastroenterology & Hepatology. děc 2004;16(12):1281-6.

65. Roos S, Karner A, Hallert C. Psychological well-being of adult coeliac patients treated for 10 years. Dig Liver Dis. March 2006;38(3):177-80.

66. Viljamaa M, Collin P, Huhtala H, Sievanen H, Maki M, Kaukinen K. Is coeliac disease screening in risk groups justified? A fourteen-year follow-up with special focus on compliance and quality of life. Aliment PharmacolTher. 15 August 2005;22(4):317-24.

67. Guennouni M, El Khoudri N, Bourrouhouate A, Hilali A. Availability and cost of gluten-free products in Moroccan supermarkets and e-commerce platforms. BFJ. 3 janv2022;124(1):1-13.

68. Pourhoseingholi MA, Rostami-Nejad M, Barzegar F, Rostami K, Volta U, Sadeghi A, et al. Economic burden made celiac disease an expensive and challenging condition for Iranian patients. GastroenterolHepatolBed Bench. 2017;10(4):258-62.

69. Reimbursement for gluten-free products [Internet]. [сИё 18 fisvr 2024]. Available from: https://www.afdiag.fr/au-quotidien/remboursement-des-produits-sans-gluten/

70. Coeliac UK [Internet]. [сИё   18 fëvr 2024]. Prescriptions. Available from: https://www.coeliac.org.uk/information-and-support/coeliac-disease/once-diagnosed/prescriptions/

71. Celiac Disease Foundation [Internet]. [сИё 18 fëvr 2024]. Policies Around the World. Available from: https://celiac.org/gluten-free-living/global-associations-and-policies/policies-around-the-world/

7 APPENDICES

❖ APPENDIX 1: Socio-demographic, anamnestic and clinical characteristics of patients

السن

الجنس □ :ذكر □ /أنثى

الحالةالمدنية □ :عازب(ة /)□متزوج(ة /)□مطلق(ة /)□ارمل(ة

المستوىالاجتماعيوالاقتصادي حسبالدخلالشهري □ :دون المتوسط(أقلمن 500 دينارفيالشهر) □متوسطبين (500 و

دينارفيالشهر)□ /فوقالمتوسط(أكثرمن 1500 دينارفيالشهر 1500

المستوىالدراسي □ :إبتدائي □ /ثانوي □ /جامعي

مكانالاقامة □ :المدينة □ /الريف

هلتدخن : □نعم □ /لا

هليعانيأحدافراد عائلتكمنهذاالمرض : □نعم □ /لا

هلتعانيمنإحدىأمراضالمناعةالذاتية □ :مرضالسكري □ /أمراضالغددالدرقية □ /مرضالتهابالكبدالمناعيالذاتي /

لأأعانيمنايمرضمناعةذاتيةآخر□

كمكانعمركلماالكتشفمرضك

ماهية مدةتطورمرضك

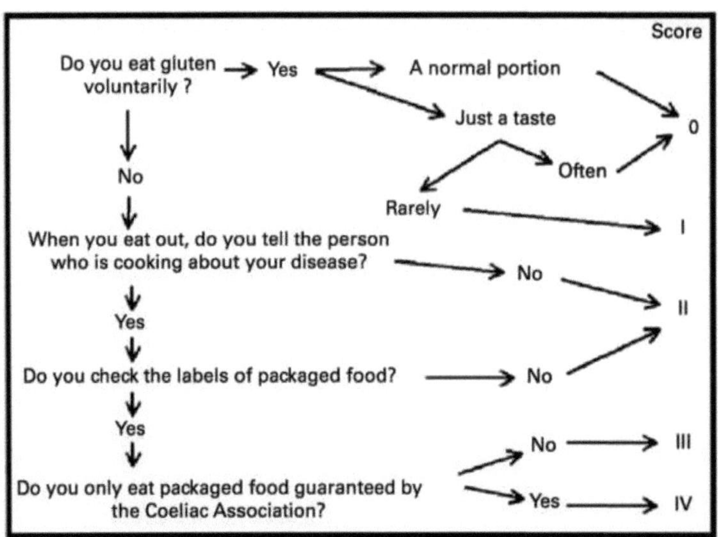

❖ *0 and I*: No follow-up by the RSG

❖ *II*: Follow-up of the RSG but with major errors that need to be corrected

❖ *III and W*: Strict monitoring of the RSG.

يدور هذا المسح حول عدد من الأسئلة والاستفسارات حول صحتك ومشاركتك هذه المعلومات التالية في متابعة حالتك الصحية ومدى قدرتك على القيام بأنشطتك اليومية.

الرجاء الإجابة على كل سؤال وذلك من خلال اختيار الإجابة المناسبة كما هو مبين، وإذا لم تكن متأكدا حول إجابة سؤال ما، فالرجاء إعطاء الإجابة الأقرب لتصحيح ما أمكن ذلك.

١- بصفة عامة يمكنك القول بأن صحتك (حالتك الصحية):

ممتازة	جيدة جدا	جيدة	حسنة	ضعيفة
☐	☐	☐	☐	☐

الأسئلة التالية تدور حول الأنشطة التي يمكنك القيام بها في يومك العادي. هل تحد حالتك الصحية الآن من هذه الأنشطة؟ إذا كانت الإجابة بنعم، إلى أي مدى؟

٢- الأنشطة المعتدلة، مثل تحريك طاولة، دفع مكنسة كهربائية، لعب الكرة.

نعم، محدودة	نعم، محدودة	لا، غير محدودة
كثيرا	قليلا	إطلاقا
☐	☐	☐

٣- صعود عدة طوابق من الدرج

| ☐ | ☐ | ☐ |

خلال الأربع أسابيع الماضية هل واجهت أي من المشاكل التالية في عملك أو في أي من نشاطاتك اليومية المنتظمة الأخرى نتيجة لحالتك الصحية؟

لا	نعم

٤- أنجزت في عملك أو نشاطاتك أقل مما كنت تصبو إليه (أو تريده).

| ☐ | ☐ |

٥- كنت محدودا في نوعية العمل أو أنشطة أخرى.

| ☐ | ☐ |

خلال الأربع أسابيع الماضية، هل واجهت أي من المشاكل التالية في عملك أو نشاطاتك اليومية المعتادة الأخرى نتيجة لأي مشاكل نفسية (أو مشاكل عاطفية مؤثرة) مثل (الشعور بالاكتئاب أو القلق)؟

لا	نعم

٦- أنجزت أقل مما كنت تصبو إليه (أو تريده أو تودّه)

| ☐ | ☐ |

٧- لم تقم بالعمل أو أنشطة أخرى بدقة (باهتمام وحذر) كالمعتاد

| ☐ | ☐ |

٨- خلال الأربع أسابيع الماضية، إلى أي مدى أثر ما تشعر به من ألم في عملك اليومي (بما في ذلك عملك خارج وداخل المنزل)

لا ألم	قليلا جدا	بصورة متوسطة	كثيرا	بشدة
☐	☐	☐	☐	☐

الأسئلة التالية تتعلق بشعورك وكيف كانت تبدو لك الأشياء خلال الأربع أسابيع الأخيرة. الرجاء إعطاء الإجابة الأقرب لما كنت تشعر به:

كم هي المدة الزمنية خلال الأربع أسابيع الماضية التي:

كل الوقت	معظم الوقت	بعض الوقت	قليلا من الوقت	لا شيء من الوقت

٩- التي شعرت فيها بالهدوء والأمن

| ☐ | ☐ | ☐ | ☐ | ☐ |

١٠- كان لديك كثيرا من الطاقة

| ☐ | ☐ | ☐ | ☐ | ☐ |

١١- هل شعرت بأي إحباط أو انكسار

| ☐ | ☐ | ☐ | ☐ | ☐ |

١٢- خلال الأربع أسابيع الأخيرة، إلى أي مدى أثرت حالتك الصحية أو النفسية في أنشطتك الاجتماعية (مثل زيارة الأقارب أو الأصدقاء إلخ)

كل الوقت	معظم الوقت	بعض الوقت	قليلا من الوقت	لا شيء من الوقت
☐	☐	☐	☐	☐

❖ **ANNEX 4: ARABIC VERSION OF THE CDQ :**

❖ 1. كم مرة خلال الأسبوعين الماضيين تأثرت حياتك بالحاجة المفاجئة لزيارة الحمام بسبب الإسهال ؟

كل الوقت 1	2 معظم الوقت	3 قدرا كبيرا من الوقت	4 بعض الوقت	5 القليل من الوقت	6 بالكاد في أي وقت	7 أبدا

❖ 2. كم مرة خلال الأسبوعين الآخرين شعرت بالإرهاق البدني أو التعب ؟

كل الوقت 1	2 معظم الوقت	3 قدرا كبيرا من الوقت	4 بعض الوقت	5 القليل من الوقت	6 بالكاد في أي وقت	7 أبدا

❖ 3. كم مرة خلال الأسبوعين الآخرين شعرت(ي) بالإحباط أو نفاذ الصبر أو الاضطراب ؟

كل الوقت 1	2 معظم الوقت	3 قدرا كبيرا من الوقت	4 بعض الوقت	5 القليل من الوقت	6 بالكاد في أي وقت	7 أبدا

❖ 4. كم عدد المرات خلال الأسبوعين الآخرين رفضت أو تجنبتدعوة لتناول العشاء مع الأصدقاء أو الأقارب بسبب مرضك بالسلياك ؟

كل الوقت 1	2 معظم الوقت	3 قدرا كبيرا من الوقت	4 بعض الوقت	5 القليل من الوقت	6 بالكاد في أي وقت	7 أبدا

❖ 5. كم مرة خلال الأسبوعين الآخرين كان لديك براز رخو؟

كل الوقت 1	2 معظم الوقت	3 قدرا كبيرا من الوقت	4 بعض الوقت	5 القليل من الوقت	6 بالكاد في أي وقت	7 أبدا

❖ 6. ما مقدار الطاقة الفكرية التي كانت لديك خلال الأسبوعين الماضيين؟

كل الوقت 1	2 معظم الوقت	3 قدرا كبيرا من الوقت	4 بعض الوقت	5 القليل من الوقت	6 بالكاد في أي وقت	7 أبدا

❖ 7. كم مرة خلال الأسبوعين الآخرين كنت تشعر(ين) بالقلق من أن أطفالك يمكن أن يرثوا أو قد ورثوا مرضك بالسلياك ؟

كل الوقت 1	2 معظم الوقت	3 قدرا كبيرا من الوقت	4 بعض الوقت	5 القليل من الوقت	6 بالكاد في أي وقت	7 أبدا

❖ 8. كم مرة خلال الأسبوعين الماضيين انزعجت من تشنجات أو مغص في بطنك؟

كل الوقت 1	2 معظم الوقت	3 قدرا كبيرا من الوقت	4 بعض الوقت	5 القليل من الوقت	6 بالكاد في أي وقت	7 أبدا

❖ 9. هل واجهت خلال الأسبوعين الآخرين أي صعوبات في الأنشطة الترفيهية أو الرياضة بسبب مرضكبالسلياك؟

كل الوقت 1	2 معظم الوقت	3 قدرا كبيرا من الوقت	4 بعض الوقت	5 القليل من الوقت	6 بالكاد في أي وقت	7 أبدا

❖ 10. كم مرة خلال الأسبوعين الآخرين كنت تشعر(ين) بالاكتئاب أو الإحباط خلال ؟

كل الوقت 1	2 معظم الوقت	3 قدرا كبيرا من الوقت	4 بعض الوقت	5 القليل من الوقت	6 بالكاد في أي وقت	7 أبدا

❖ 11. كم مرة خلال الأسبوعين الآخرين كنت تعاني (ين)من تورم أو انتفاخ البطن ؟

كل الوقت 1	2 معظم الوقت	3 قدرا كبيرا من الوقت	4 بعض الوقت	5 القليل من الوقت	6 بالكاد في أي وقت	7 أبدا

❖ 12. الناس الذين يعانون من مرض السيلياك أو الاضطرابات الهضمية غالبا ما يكون لديهم مخاوف وتوجسات متعلقة بمرضهم. كم مرة خلال الأسبوعين الآخرين كنتقلق(ة) أو خائف(ة) من الإصابة بالسرطان كنتيجة لمرضك بالسيلياك ؟

كل الوقت 1	2 معظم الوقت	3 قدرا كبيرا من الوقت	4 بعض الوقت	5 القليل من الوقت	6 بالكاد في أي وقت	7 أبدا

❖ 13. كم مرة خلال الأسبوعين الآخرين تأثرت بشعور تفريغ الأمعاء غير المكتمل ؟

كل الوقت 1	2 معظم الوقت	3 قدرا كبيرا من الوقت	4 بعض الوقت	5 القليل من الوقت	6 بالكاد في أي وقت	7 أبدا

❖ 14. كم مرة خلال الأسبوعين الآخرين شعرتبالاسترخاء وعدم التوتر؟

كل الوقت 1	2 معظم الوقت	3 قدرا كبيرا من الوقت	4 بعض الوقت	5 القليل من الوقت	6 بالكاد في أي وقت	7 أبدا

❖ 15. كم مرة خلال الأسبوعين الأخيرين شعرتبالعزلة أو الإقصاء من قبل الآخرين بسبب مرضك بالسيلياك؟

كل الوقت 1	2 معظم الوقت	3 قدرا كبيرا من الوقت	4 بعض الوقت	5 القليل من الوقت	6 بالكاد في أي وقت	7 أبدا

❖ 16. كم من الوقت خلال الأسبوعين الأخيرين شعرت بالدموع أو الغضب؟

كل الوقت 1	2 معظم الوقت	3 قدرا كبيرا من الوقت	4 بعض الوقت	5 القليل من الوقت	6 بالكاد في أي وقت	7 أبدا

❖ 17. كم مرة خلال الأسبوعين الماضيين عانيت من التجشؤ المتكرر؟

كل الوقت 1	2 معظم الوقت	3 قدرا كبيرا من الوقت	4 بعض الوقت	5 القليل من الوقت	6 بالكاد في أي وقت	7 أبدا

❖ 18. إلى أي مدى خلال الأسبوعين الآخرين قيّد مرض السيلياك نشاطك الجنسي ؟

كل الوقت 1	2 معظم الوقت	3 قدرا كبيرا من الوقت	4 بعض الوقت	5 القليل من الوقت	6 بالكاد في أي وقت	7 أبدا

❖ 19. كم مرة خلال الأسبوعين الماضيين عانيت من الغثيان أو محاولة التقيء؟

كل الوقت 1	2 معظم الوقت	3 قدرا كبيرا من الوقت	4 بعض الوقت	5 القليل من الوقت	6 بالكاد في أي وقت	7 أبدا

❖ 20. كم مرة خلال الأسبوعين الأخيرين شعرت أن أشخاص مهمين مثل أفراد عائلتك أو أصدقائك أبانوا عن عدم فهم لمرضك بالسيلياك؟

7 أبدا	6 بالكاد في أي وقت	5 القليل من الوقت	4 بعض الوقت	3 قدرا كبيرا من الوقت	2 معظم الوقت	كل الوقت 1

❖ 21. ما مدى رضاك أو سعادتك أو انبساطك في حياتك الشخصية خلال الأسبوعين الماضيين؟

7 أبدا	6 بالكاد في أي وقت	5 القليل من الوقت	4 بعض الوقت	3 قدرا كبيرا من الوقت	2 معظم الوقت	كل الوقت 1

❖ 22. كم مرة خلال الأسبوعين الأخيرين شعرتأن الزملاء أو الرؤساء أبانوا عن عدم فهم لمرضك بالسيلياك؟

7 أبدا	6 بالكاد في أي وقت	5 القليل من الوقت	4 بعض الوقت	3 قدرا كبيرا من الوقت	2 معظم الوقت	كل الوقت 1

❖ 23. كم مرة خلال الأسبوعين الماضيين شعرت بمحدوديتك في التدريب المهني أو في وظيفتك بسبب مرضك بالسيلياك ؟

7 أبدا	6 بالكاد في أي وقت	5 القليل من الوقت	4 بعض الوقت	3 قدرا كبيرا من الوقت	2 معظم الوقت	كل الوقت 1

❖ 24. كم مرة خلال الأسبوعين الأخيرين شعرت أن صعوبة الحصول على طعام خالٍ من الغلوتين تثقل كاهلك؟

7 أبدا	6 بالكاد في أي وقت	5 القليل من الوقت	4 بعض الوقت	3 قدرا كبيرا من الوقت	2 معظم الوقت	كل الوقت 1

❖ 25. كم مرة خلال الأسبوعين الأخيرين شعرتأن المشاكل المتعلقة بتمويل الأطعمة الخالية من الغلوتين أو غيرها من علاج الاضطرابات الهضمية (على سبيل المثال ، التكاليف ، والوصفات الطبية ، و التعويضات) تثقل كاهلك؟

7 أبدا	6 بالكاد في أي وقت	5 القليل من الوقت	4 بعض الوقت	3 قدرا كبيرا من الوقت	2 معظم الوقت	كل الوقت 1

❖ 26. كم عدد المرات خلال الأسبوعين الماضيين عانيت من نقص الخبرة في مرض السيلياك من طرف أطبائك؟

1 كل الوقت	2 معظم الوقت	3 قدرا كبيرا من الوقت	4 بعض الوقت	5 القليل من الوقت	6 بالكاد في أي وقت	7 أبدا

❖ 27. كم مرة خلال الأسبوعين الماضيين كنتقلقا (ة) من أن مرض السيلياك تم تشخيصه بعد فوات الأوان؟

1 كل الوقت	2 معظم الوقت	3 قدرا كبيرا من الوقت	4 بعض الوقت	5 القليل من الوقت	6 بالكاد في أي وقت	7 أبدا

❖ 28. كم مرة خلال الأسبوعين الماضيين عانيت من الخوف من الفحوصات الطبية فيما يتعلق بمرض السيلياك ، على سبيل المثال سحب الدم أو المنظار الباطني

1 كل الوقت	2 معظم الوقت	3 قدرا كبيرا من الوقت	4 بعض الوقت	5 القليل من الوقت	6 بالكاد في أي وقت	7 أبدا

1. In general, would you say your health is:	
Excellent	1
Very good	2
Good	3
Fair	4
Poor	5
2. Compared to one year ago,	
Much better now than one year ago	1
Somewhat better now than one year ago	2
About the same	3
Somewhat worse now than one year ago	4
Much worse now than one year ago	5

3. The following items are about activities you might do during a typical day. Does your health now limit you in these activities? If so, how much?

(Circle One Number on Each Line)

	Yes, Limited a Lot (1)	Yes, Limited a Little (2)	No, Not limited at All (3)
a. **Vigorous activities,** such as running, lifting heavy objects, participating in strenuous sports	1	2	3
b. **Moderate activities,** such as moving a table, pushing a vacuum cleaner, bowling, or playing golf	1	2	3
c. Lifting or carrying groceries	1	2	3
d. Climbing **several** flights of stairs	1	2	3
e. Climbing **one** flight of stairs	1	2	3
f. Bending, kneeling, or stooping	1	2	3
g. Walking **more than a mile**	1	2	3
h. Walking **several blocks**	1	2	3
i. Walking **one block**	1	2	3
j. Bathing or dressing yourself	1	2	3

4. During the **past 4 weeks,** have you had any of the following problems with your work or other regular daily activities **as a result of your physical health?**

(Circle One Number on Each Line)

	Yes (1)	No (2)

a. Cut down the amount of time you spent on work or other activities	1	2
b. **Accomplished less** than you would like	1	2
c. Were limited in the **kind of** work or other activities	1	2
d. Had **difficulty** performing the work or other activities (for example, it took extra effort)	1	2

5.   During the **past 4 weeks,** have you had any of the following problems with your work or other regular daily activities **as a result of any emotional problems** (such as feeling depressed or anxious)?

(Circle One Number on Each Line)

	Yes	No
a. Cut down the amount of time you spent on work or other activities	1	2
b. **Accomplished less** than you would like	1	2
c. Didn't do work or other activities as **carefully** as usual	1	2
6. During the past 4 weeks, to what extent has your physical health or emotional problems interfered with your normal social activities with family, friends, neighbors, or groups?		
Not at all	1	
Slightly	2	
Moderately	3	
Quite a bit	4	
Extremely	5	
7. How much bodily pain have you had during the past 4 weeks?		
None	1	
Very mild	2	
Mild	3	
Moderate	4	
Severe	5	
Very severe	6	
8. During the past 4 weeks, how much did pain interfere with your normal work (including both work outside the home and housework)?		
Not at all	1	
A little bit	2	
Moderately	3	
Quite a bit	4	
Extremely	5	

These questions are about how you feel and how things have been with you **during the past 4 weeks.** For each question, please give the one answer that comes closest to the way you have been feeling **(Circle One Number on Each Line).**

9. How much of the time during the **past 4 weeks**

	AU of the Time	Most of the Time	A Good Bit of the Time	Some of the Time	A Little of the Time	None of the Time
a. Did you feel full of pep?	1	2	3	4	5	6
b. Have you been a very nervous person?	1	2	3	4	5	6
c. Have you felt so down in the dumps that nothing could cheer you up?	1	2	3	4	5	6
d. Have you felt calm and peaceful?	1	2	3	4	5	6
e. Did you have a lot of energy?	1	2	3	4	5	6
	All of the Time	Most of the Time	A Good Bit of the Time	Some of the Time	A Little of the Time	None of the Time
f. Have you felt downhearted and blue?	1	2	3	4	5	6
g. Did you feel worn out?	1	2	3	4	5	6
h. Have you been a happy person?	1	2	3	4	5	6
i. Did you feel tired?	1	2	3	4	5	6

10. During the past 4 weeks, how much of the time has your physical health or emotional problems interfered with your social activities (like visiting with friends, relatives, etc.)? (Circle One Number)

All of the time	1
Most of the time	2
Some of the time	3
A little of the time	4
None of the time	5

11. How TRUE or FALSE is each of the following statements for you (Circle One Number on Each Line)

	Definitely True	Mostly True	Don't Know	Mostly False	Definitely False
a. I seem to get sick a little easier than other people	1	2	3	4	5
b. I am as healthy as anybody I know	1	2	3	4	5
c. I expect my health to get worse	1	2	3	4	5
d. My health is excellent	1	2	3	4	5

Score	Anxiety	Score	Depression
	I feel tense or nervous:		I take pleasure in the same things I used to
3	□ most of the time	0	□ yes, just as much
2	□ often	1	□ not so much
1	□ from time to time	2	□ just a little
0	□ never	3	□ almost no more
	I have a feeling of fear as if something something horrible was going to happen to me		I laugh easily and look on the bright side.
		0	□ as much as the past
3	□ yes, very clearly	1	□ not as much as before
2	□ yes, but it doesn't matter	2	□ really less than before
1	□ a little, but that doesn't worry me	3	□ not at all
0	□ not at all		
	I'm worried:		I'm in a good mood:
3	□ very often	3	□ never
2	□ quite often	2	□ rarely
1	□ occasionally	1	□ quite often
0	□ very occasionally	0	□ most of the time
	I рейх to sit quietly doing nothing and feel relaxed:		I feel like I'm idling:
		3	□ almost always
0	□ yes, whatever happens	2	□ very often
1	□ yes, in general	1	□ sometimes
2	□ rarely	0	□ never
3	□ never		
	I have a feeling of fear and my stomach is in knots. knot:		I'm no longer interested in my appearance:
		3	□ not at all
0	□ never	2	□ I don't pay as much attention to it as I should
1	□ sometimes		□ I may not pay as much attention to it anymore
2	□ quite often	1	□ I pay as much attention to it as I did in the past
3	□ very often	0	
	I'm restless and can't keep still: □ yes, that's absolutely the case		I'm looking forward to doing certain things: П as much as before
3	□ a little	0	□ a little less than before
2	□ not tenement	1	□ much less than before
1	□ not at all	2	□ almost never
0		3	
	I have sudden feelings of panic: □ very often		I рейх take pleasure in a good book or a good radio or television broadcast :
3	□ quite often	0	□ often
2	□ not very often	1	□ sometimes
1	□ never	2	□ rarely
0		3	□ very rarely
	■® Total anxiety score		Total depression score

Each response corresponds to a number. Adding these numbers together gives a total score per column (anxiëtë and dëpression). If the score for a column is greater than or ёдаl to 11, this means that you suffer from anxiëtë or dëpression (depending on the column concerned).

APPENDIX 7:QuestionnaireCD-QOL

CD-QOL Scale (final version) CD-QOL Survey

Please think about your life over the past month (30 days), and look at the statements below. Each statement has five possible responses. For each statement, please fill in one box in each row that best describes your feelings.

	Not at all 1	Slightly 2	Moderately 3	Quite a bit 4	A great deal 5
1 I feel limited by this disease	☐	☐	☐	☐	☐
2 I feel worried that I will suffer from this disease	☐	☐	☐	☐	☐
3 I feel concerned that this disease will cause other health problems	☐	☐	☐	☐	☐
4 I feel worried about my increased risk of cancer from this disease	☐	☐	☐	☐	☐
5 I feel socially stigmatised for having this disease.	☐	☐	☐	☐	☐
6 I feel like I'm limited in eating meals with coworkers	☐	☐	☐	☐	☐
7 I feel like I am not able to have special foods like birthday cake and pizza	☐	☐	☐	☐	☐
8 I feel that the diet is sufficient treatment for my disease	☐	☐	☐	☐	☐
9 I feel that there are not enough choices for treatment	☐	☐	☐	☐	☐
10 I feel depressed because of my disease	☐	☐	☐	☐	☐
11 I feel frightened by having this disease	☐	☐	☐	☐	☐
12 I feel like I don't know enough about the disease	☐	☐	☐	☐	☐
13 I feel overwhelmed about having this disease	☐	☐	☐	☐	☐
14 I have trouble socializing because of my disease	☐	☐	☐	☐	☐
15 I find it difficult to travel or take long trips because of my disease	☐	☐	☐	☐	☐
16 I feel like I cannot live a normal life because of my disease	☐	☐	☐	☐	☐
17 I feel afraid to eat out because my food may be contaminated	☐	☐	☐	☐	☐
18 I feel worried about the increased risk of one of my family members having coeliac disease	☐	☐	☐	☐	☐
19 I feel like I think about food all the time	☐	☐	☐	☐	☐
20 I feel concerned that my long-term health will be affected	☐	☐	☐	☐	☐

Evaluation of the quality of life in patients with a

TITLE Calia disease

Introduction: Celiac disease (CD) is an autoimmune disorder whose influence on patients' quality of life (QoL) is multidimensional, which is why its evaluation is so important.

The aim of this study was to assess the quality of life of patients with CD and to determine the factors associated with its deterioration.

Method: We conducted a descriptive and analytical cross-sectional study over a three-month period from 1 October to 31 December 2023, including 100 patients who were members of the Tunisian Celiac Disease Association. QOL was assessed using two valid questionnaires available in Arabic: a general questionnaire (the SF-12) and a questionnaire specific to CD (the creliacdisease questionnaire (CDQ)).

Results: We included 100 patients, with a mean age of 34.5 ± 9.5 years and a sex ratio (males/females) of 0.39:1. The median age at disease onset was 11 years [IIQ= 2-30] with a median duration of 21.5 years [IIQ= 6.25-28]. Evaluation of adherence to the gluten-free diet revealed that 73 patients (73%) did not adhere to a strict GFD.

The mean SF-12 total score was 26.00 ± 4.01. All patients had scores below 40, for the global score as well as for the mental and physical components, corresponding to an altered QoL. Specific assessment by the CDQ resulted in a mean global score of 123.86 ± 29.57 out of a maximum score of 196. In univariate analysis, the factors associated with an altered QOL according to the SF-12 were: female gender (p=0.02), non-university education (p<0.001), and history of associated autoimmune diseases (p=0.04). Those according to the CDQ were: low NSE (p=0.01), non-university education (p=0.02) and the presence of personal history of autoimmune diseases (p=0.02).

The independent factors identified after adjustment were: non-university education level (Beta=0.21; p=0.03; 95% CI [0.10; 3.59]) with the SF-12 and low NSE (Beta=0.25; p=0.04; 95% CI [1.05; 42.50]) with the CDQ.

Conclusion:

CD significantly affects patients' quality of life. Poor educational and socio-economic status contribute more to this impairment. These data open up prospects for psychotherapeutic intervention in patients with CD, with the aim of improving their quality of life as part of comprehensive, personalised care.

KEYWORDS Celiac Disease / Quality Of Life / SF12 / CD-QUESTIONNAIRE

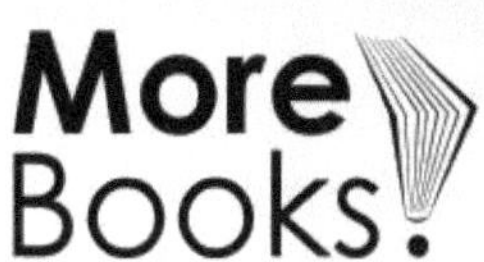

More
Books!

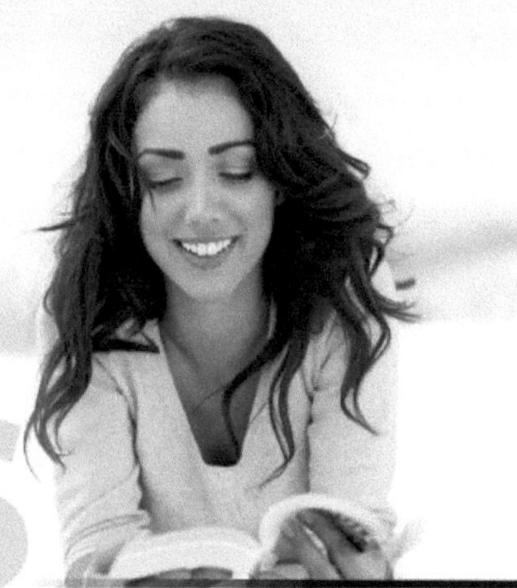

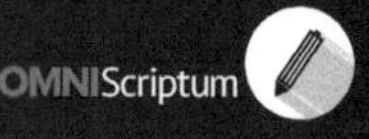

info@omniscriptum.com
www.omniscriptum.com
OMNIScriptum

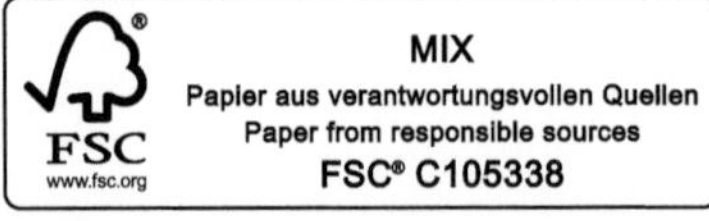

Printed by Books on Demand GmbH, Norderstedt / Germany